FORCED TO FOCUS

FORCED TO FOCUS

A PASTOR'S FAITH JOURNEY THROUGH CANCER

Ronald L. Griffin

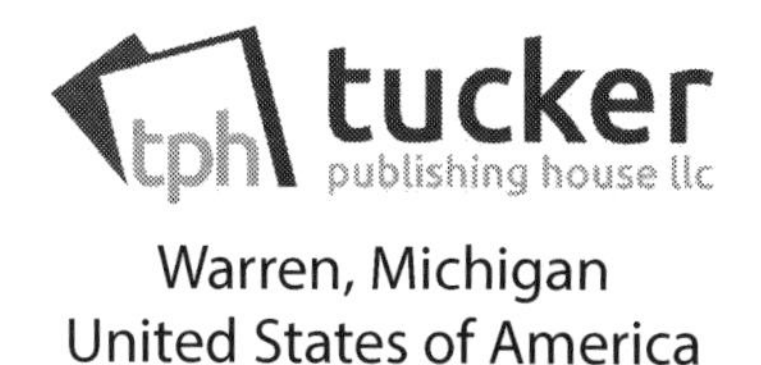

Warren, Michigan
United States of America

"This book will serve as a self-help manual for people who are faced with cancer or other ailments. His testimony will inspire others to trust God for their healing, stay in faith, keep a positive outlook and energy as they travel their journey of healing. This book will encourage you to get to know God in a more intimate way. It will enlighten and encourage you to keep pressing forward in every area of your life."

-Mother Kendra Ford-

"This book will be an inspiring book to read. I feel this book is a look into a Pastor's life as he goes through a rare form of cancer. Christians are often looked at as people that don't go through anything; people who often can't relate to today's problems. This book gives an up close and personal look into the life of a person who is human and nonexempt from the world that we live in. This book shows how just because you are religious, you are still human, and you have the same problems. It tells the emotional roller coaster this man of GOD has gone through during his fight against cancer. This book goes into every single detail of a Pastor's life from beginning to end on all his feelings and emotions. I feel this book will inspire, encourage, and reach souls who might be going through the same fight and need to know

they are not alone. This book will inspire you to keep fighting, keep believing, and to have faith."

-Sister Zequetta Hall-

This was not just a book, but a POWERFUL testimony of how a GREAT MAN OF GOD executed the scripture, "For we walk by Faith, not by sight" (2 Corinthians 5:7) during his cancer journey. Reading this book is bound to inspire, motivate, and empower every reader that touches it, because the same God that did it for him can do it for all of us; He's just that POWERFUL!!

-Regina D. Coleman-

Founder of Saving Our Sisters by Knowing My Truth Nonprofit Organization

Forced to Focus

 Scriptures, unless
otherwise noted, were taken from the King James Version (KJV.)

First edition, Author Ronald L. Griffin

Paperback ISBN: 978-1-7377140-6-4

Library of Congress Number: 2021925876

Published 2021 by

Tucker Publishing House, LLC

Warren, Michigan

www.tuckerpublishinghouse.com

Published in the United States of America

Dedication

Upon reflection of those to whom I would honor in the dedication of "*Forced to Focus*" it became very clear that I owe the following people so much:

My parents, Richard & Vivian Clowney and Bishop Willie L. & Mother Ima Harris. Throughout my life my mother & father, nurtured, encouraged, cajoled, pushed, chastised, and forced me to focus on the ability, talent, and skills that God gave me. They always, without fail, emphasized that I could do anything that I put my mind to do. I was raised in the church, and taught, "right from wrong."

They sacrificed everything for me and my sister, Joyce. I miss them right now and, I know that they would be very proud of my accomplishments. I recall on one occasion I said to them, "If I am successful in life, you will get all the credit and if I'm a failure, I'll take all the blame."

For my "in-laws," my mother & father-in-law were the absolute best of the best. They treated me more like I was their biological son, not just joined together by marriage to their daughter. They set such an impressive example of what true holiness and Christ like people should be. From day one, Mother Harris saw my future. She commented to Linda, "The Ron you see today is not the Ron you'll see tomorrow." Bishop Harris saw a mirror image of himself in some instances and treated me accordingly; they too would be proud of me.

Now, the most wonderful, perfect wife, friend, and soul mate that I am so grateful for, Linda F. Griffin, my wife of 50 years. She has always stood by my side comforting me in times of distress, encouraging me to continue to go forward and loving me unconditionally. Linda accompanied me throughout my cancer journey and was the first to say to me, "Write the book. Tell your story. Give your testimony." She was with me during the surgery, when we got the Pathologists report, "It's 3rd stage cancer" and at every radiation treatment. All of this and so much more. It is because of her, our parents, and all to God's glory that "*Forced to Focus*" became a reality. I cannot thank God enough for what they are in my life.

TABLE OF CONTENTS

Foreword

I am Mrs. Linda F. Griffin, the wife of the author. I am a true Believer in Jesus Christ and His Healing Power. I am the ninth child born to the late Bishop Willie Leroy and Mother Ima Mae Harris. I am the mother of two adult children and the grandmother of eight. I am a graduate of Wayne State University and the First Lady of Rose of Sharon Church of God in Christ, located in Detroit, Michigan.

Now with that being said—I love, respect, and admire the author of this book. He has captured my heart, and down through the years (fifty of them) I have come to realize that we have fought and survived so many earthly and spiritual battles together to the Glory of God.

It was in the 49th year of our marriage that tragedy struck: The cancer journey; and I was "*Forced to Focus.*" My faith, marriage vows, and our finances were put to the ultimate test, and I was looking at the final chapter of my dear husband's existence. I was forced to depend on God for all of the answers. You notice that I didn't put my faith in his attending physicians, because at the end of the day, God directs all medical professionals—no matter how much education and scientific knowledge they've attained.

It must be known to the reader of this book that I stood tall, never complained, and constantly went to church and bible study, while asking God in prayer—"IS THIS HOW OUR STORY WILL END?

Believe me Reader, you will be challenged by God Almighty with a test; and while He knows how the story will end, He is waiting on your involvement. Will you stand, or will you fold up? It is up to you to write your ending, and truly depend on God to do the rest.

In conclusion, the author, The Right Reverend Ronald L. Griffin, is truly a man of God and a mighty man of faith. He doesn't just *say* he believes in God; he has lived it before me, his family, friends, and congregation.

He was absolutely "*Forced to Focus*" on God after a four-hour surgery to remove a tumor that was 6 cc (3 inches) and a horrific and frightening diagnosis of 3rd Stage Cancer) an agonizing and expensive trip to Zion Illinois (Cancer Treatment Center of America) only to find out they agreed with the first diagnosis. Next, was a daily regiment for seven grueling long weeks (thirty-three radiation treatments to the face, ear and throat). Our collective faith in God was challenged.

Finally, Reader, God's Word is true. As promised by our Lord and Savior Jesus Christ, in the time of trouble "He will hide you in a secret place where the enemy can't find or harm you." Today, my husband, pastor, father of two children and grandfather of eight, is cancer free, and is truly focused on the next chapter of his life. Be assured that no matter the test, or the bumpy journey, God never promised that the road to heaven would be without challenges. However, He did say that He would provide a safe landing after the ride. He will always provide a path with a directional map for you to follow. Please enjoy reading this heartfelt book, as you are faced with your own life changes and challenges.

Mrs. Linda F. Griffin

Introduction

The purpose of sharing my cancer journey and testimony is twofold. First and of utmost importance, I want to encourage believers and non-believers to trust God and know that he has the answer to all of life's trials and tribulations. He has the answer because *He is the answer!*

Allow me to explain it this way. I attended a "Homegoing Service" for a great man of God who, when the Eulogist finished his message, we were left with three emotions; 1.) I wished I would have known the man; 2.) I knew him but wished I would have gotten to know him better; 3.) I'm so glad that he was a good friend of mine. As you read "*Forced to Focus*", I want you to fall into one of those three categories. I want you to experience a renewed focus of your own to know that our Lord and Savior Jesus Christ is a healer and deliverer, no matter what's going on in our lives and in the world in which we exist.

Secondly, I've had many opportunities to pray for individuals that were diagnosed with some form of cancer. I prayed the prayer of faith and honestly felt deep concern and compassion for the afflicted; but now that I am experiencing my own cancer journey, I have an up-close and personal viewpoint that has changed my ministry forever. My heart goes out with a deeper respect to all those who have survived cancer and a greater understanding of their faith, bravery, prayer life, and desire to stand tall in the face of such a devastating health challenge. It is because of my own journey that I will continue to approach and support the families whose loved ones succumbed to its devastation and went on to be with the Lord.

Now, before I offer condolences, I will ask "What can I do to help you?" or "What do you need me to do?" My hope and prayer is that this book will give you profound insight on what I experienced and help you to see, you are not alone. I want born-again believers and servants of the Most High God to realize what a blessing it is to be chosen by Him for His Glory.

Immediately after I was diagnosed with Stage 3 Cancer, the Lord spoke to me in the Spirit and said, *"Everyone says they want to be more like me, but no one wants to suffer or make sacrifices like I did. So, how can you become more like me if you are reluctant to walk the same pathways I walked."* And that conversation prepared me for the journey and ultimately this book, "*Forced to Focus.*"

So, we look to all the usual or familiar resources for direction instead of placing our focus on God. The politicians and the parties they represent are divided and largely dysfunctional and popular talk show hosts and so-called current events analysts are "clueless" with no personal experience that would connect them with the human conditions. The Religious community who should be setting the example for civility, forgiveness, Godly love, compassion, and spiritual unity have, in my opinion, become instruments used by special interest groups pushing their own agenda. We, the clergy, can't seem to agree on anything except perhaps that God is real and even that declaration is contaminated by our own self-developed theology in too many instances.

Social justice has historically and rampantly become social *injustice.* Even while protestors marched, people were not only denied their constitutional rights, protection, and privilege; the killings and injustice often continued with no recompense. There are so many more examples that I could use; however, I believe you get the point. Given the above scenario, I firmly believe the almighty God is "doing His best" to get our attention.

Examine, if you will, the contamination of the Pandemic: division and violence over Vaccination vs Non-Vaccination; Mask vs No Mask; Global warming; Anti-abortion vs. Life choice; Social unrest and senseless violence. Bias media in all forms are fueling the flames in every strata of society and dysfunction in our families. So then, it is my assignment to use my personal experience during my cancer journey to encourage you.

"*Forced to Focus*" has given me a clearer picture and a closer relationship with Him to know that He is The Answer. In the face of what sometimes seems like there is no answer and no way out of this horrible place, we must return to Him! He said in his word at 2 Chronicles 7:14, "If my people, which are called by my name, shall humble themselves, and pray, and seek my face, and turn from their wicked ways; then will I hear from heaven and will forgive their sin, and will heal their land." It is that scripture passage that forced me to focus on Him, and it's my heart's desire that what I've experienced will encourage you to also *refocus* on Him because He is The Answer!!

Pastor Ronald L. Griffin

Chapter One

Forced to Focus

I really didn't need people to tell me that God could heal me of cancer; nor did I need people giving me pep talks. My mind was already made up and I was sure GOD was going to heal my body and allow me to testify of His goodness and what He had done for me. But what I appreciated the most was when people called and said, "I heard about your situation; what do you need me to do for you?" and then they just started praying. That's what resonated with me the most, and I felt their prayers. I needed those people that had been through something to stand in the gap and pray for me.

I didn't take my illness lightly, but I knew God was letting me know, "Now, you are going to need me more than you ever could imagine you would." Unquestionably, it was no more business as usual. I believe all of those trials and tribulations led up to God saying, "Ok, I'm going to get your attention this time for real, my servant."

I heard many people get up in the church and testify about how the doctors found a spot on their lungs, and they went back, and it was gone, and the church started shouting. Now, I didn't bother them about this because I don't question anybody if that is their testimony, but God was not going to get any glory out of ME with that same testimony. You see, if that was my experience then that meant I didn't go through any suffering or anything. Please understand it's not that I believe God can't work a miracle, but I never thought that God was going to do anything like that for me. And this may sound crazy, but I didn't ask God to heal me in this context because I didn't mind being chosen. However, this was more than a notion even when I knew God was going to heal me, He let me know you're going to feel this.

When I was first diagnosed, I wasn't in any pain. After the surgery, I stayed overnight, and the nurses said, "we're going to get the wheelchair for you" and

I said, "you can get the wheelchair for someone that can't walk." And I walked out of the hospital. I didn't start to feel anything until He told me what was about to happen. When He took my appetite and my ability to taste and swallow food, He said, "now you're really going to understand because I am going to take you to a place that you've never been before," and he started giving me scriptures.

In your personal lives, Some things spiritually you've just blown off. You've dealt with it and said thank you, Lord, and kept on moving. But you've had some other things where you've said Ok. I am going to tell you now God has something else depending upon what you need from him.

Now allow me to take you to the year of 2009. I had a great need to seek God's direction and intervention. The Rose of Sharon COGIC, the church where I have been blessed to Pastor for nearly 30 years, and my immediate family were experiencing life's trials and tribulations. The hardships took us away from our faith and depending on His word. I began to petition the Lord in earnestly believing the Word to "pray without ceasing" as it says at 1 Thessalonians 5:17. Such Prayer brought an immediate response. He replied, "What sacrifice are you willing to make if I answer your prayers?" While I was contemplating my answer, walking in the quiet solitude of the woods on our property. He continued, "give of yourself through fasting and prayer" I replied immediately, both audibly and in the spirit, "I will do it, Dear Lord." The first Sunday following my encounter, I testified, notifying the entire congregation and my family of the direction and command from the Lord.

I shut in that Monday morning, vowing to remain in solitude, fasting, praying and reading His word—committing to staying there until He released me. I avoided all contact with the "outside world;" no television, radio, social media, newspapers, or phone (only) to reassure my wife that I was okay. Each day and night, I made a point of being in the sanctuary where I could receive all that He had for me. During the day the sun would fill the sanctuary with a ray so bright that I could not look directly into it. There was a peace, an aura so awesome that I would break out in anointed praise and worship to our God. And at night, when my body needed rest, I made an "old school pallet" and slept on the floor at the altar, absorbing even the Spirit of God while I slept. "Oh, my Lord, what an experience!"

During my time with the Lord, I invited the entire church and my family to join me. Some did briefly—

mostly, not all. The Lord spoke to me, saying, "Don't be discouraged. You are the leader. Stand in for them." The fasting (soup and juice once daily, nothing after 6 pm) lasted six days and five nights before the Lord released me. I was so refreshed and energized that I felt as though I could tackle the world's problems. I was ready to call for a "Worldwide Revival." It appeared everything was headed in the right direction; victory was at hand! But little did I know, over a nineyear stretch, my church, my family, and myself endured trials and tribulations, that in essence, God was using to prepare me for the place I find myself in today "*Forced to Focus*".

Chapter Two

The Journey Begins

Let's fast forward to April 6, 2021; I began to notice what appeared to be a slight swelling on the left side of my face between my ear and jaw. Over the next few weeks, I noticed the swelling getting larger and hardening into a lump; however, I was not particularly alarmed. I knew I should have it examined by the doctors at the John D. Dingell Veteran Affairs Medical Center (I served in the United States Armed Forces, honorably discharged in 1969—4 years of service). After the examination (biopsy), the lump was diagnosed as a benign Warthin tumor. It's described in medical terms as a benign cystic tumor of the salivary glands. It is almost never malignant and can be treated without surgery. I was led to take the surgery option because the tumor was growing and getting harder to the touch.

The surgery was scheduled for May 24, 2021 and was only supposed to last about two or three hours at the longest. After nearly four hours, the mass (3 inches diameter) of the parotid gland (saliva gland) was removed. They released me to go home after an overnight stay. Thirty days later, we were advised that the pathologist's report was finished. As we waited to be told the results, my wonderful, spirit-led wife of 50 years said, "Honey, it's not going to be good." Her words were not cryptic or overly emotional. God gave us a calming peace to get ready for what was to come. Upon receipt of the results, the report indicated the mass was malignant, and I was diagnosed with Stage 3 cancer. The doctor's, I think, expected some type of emotional reaction from us, but Linda and I were in the comforting and secure hands of the Lord. I asked confidently, "What are the next steps?" "Find it and let's get it fixed," I added. I believe in medical science along with an abiding faith in the healing power of God; The doctors recommended 30 radiation treatments.

After we left the hospital, we prayed to seek the Lord's direction. How and when should we tell the family, the church, close friends, and who should we tell first? We informed the family first, our son, daughter, daughter-in-law, and five of our eight grandchildren; of course, it was a shock to them. As their father and grandfather, they had never known me to be seriously ill or "down" for anything. The very "speaking" of cancer diagnosis caused fear to overcome reason and faith. They were stunned, to say the least—tears flowed from some, while others were just numb. We experienced a similar reaction from the membership and from close personal friends. The Holy Spirit took charge with words of comfort to the family, church members, and friends. I spoke with assurance and a strong belief that I was chosen by God to do a "great work" for Him like He used Job. I felt that God trusted me to carry out His Assignment. All of this was for His Glory. I had no fear, no doubt, and no real concern. In fact, I would state, "If you see me in a fight with a bear, pour the honey on me and help the bear." You see, I lift my eyes to the hills from which cometh my help, my help cometh from the Lord, the Maker of Heaven and Earth. He will not permit thy foot to be moved, He that keepeth thee will not slumber. (Psalm 121:1-3)

This was not boastful nor vain and foolish utterances, but my sincere desire to encourage those who loved me and were dependent on my faith and strength. I wanted all of them to know we serve a God that cannot fail. I fervently wanted my testimony to inspire people to renew their relationship with our Lord and Savior, Jesus Christ. And there's more….

As I was relishing where I was with the Lord, He again spoke to me in the Spirit, uttering these words, "You and others—born again believers like to say, I want to be more like Jesus, or help me to become more Christ-like—a better Christian. Yet very few want to suffer or sacrifice as I did. How can you become more like me if you're not willing to go through as I went through?" That "sobered" me up, thus putting me into a more focused frame of mind. How willing was I to suffer and sacrifice through this cancer journey in a way that would please the Messiah? In all of this, He was not finished with me.

The Daily Touch

In the beginning, it didn't bother me simply to lose weight, except while I was losing the weight, I began to look physically at my body. For years I always received compliments that I didn't look my age but the more

I looked at my body, I saw I was losing muscle mass and I saw what they call 'creped skin wrinkles' and flesh hanging. It was at that time the Lord spoke to me and said, "All you've experienced was vanity and you used to think ain't I wonderful' but look at you now." All I saw was a wreck. During that time my wife tried to comfort me by saying, "Honey, it is going to be alright." But all I saw was the naked truth. If you want to know the depth of my feelings; first, I believed it wasn't anything. Then I heard the enemy say, "You will never be able to taste again or digest food. You will always be on a liquid diet." Well, I knew God promised to heal me, but the thought crossed my mind… It started out in the realm of possibility or probability. *Maybe I will be on a liquid diet for the rest of my life?* That is why I needed a daily touch from the Lord.

I have a number of tailor-made clothes. I looked in the closet, and none of them fit. When I looked at that, the Lord once again brought the issue of vanity to me, saying, "Why do you need all those suits; why do you need color coordinated suits with shirts, ties and shoes? You don't need it because what I'm going to do for you, none of that will be necessary. I am getting ready to redo you. Redo your thinking, your mindset, your relationship with me and your relationship with the Word." This is why every time I reached a different level in my journey; He would give me more of the Word to encourage my soul. When I wanted to eat, *He said "Man shall not live by bread alone" (Matthew 4:4)*. When I was concerned about how I looked, He reminded me it was all vanity. He then gave me the scripture, *"Trust in the Lord with all thine heart and lean not to thine own understanding and all thy ways acknowledge him, and He shall direct your path."* (Proverbs 3:5-6) He then told me to trust Him without question. Regardless of what I see and feel, I had to know He's got me, and He was going to deliver me from this.

I never thought I would die or anything like that, but it was a daily challenge. And if you have never really been through anything, you don't understand a daily walk. We say we understand it, but we take each day for granted. Every day was a different journey and I often wondered what was going to happen next? *What am I going to do?* Not only could I not taste or digest food, but because of the loss of my parotid gland, my mouth got so dry. The poison of the radiation being in my mouth caused me not to want to swallow water. You can check this; you don't know anyone that has lived off less than 500 calories per day and still physically walked, drove, worked, and gave everything. God said, "I am greater than any physical thing than you can imagine. I will sustain you when you don't eat anything for days." He reminded me that for years He had been calling me to go on a fast. He said, "Now this is a forced fast and I will fix it where you will eat nothing, and some days you won't even want to taste the water." That was my reality for over forty days.

A Blessing in Disguise

When I couldn't eat anything, my wife said, "Let's try protein shakes." That didn't work. Then we tried sugar-free jello, and that didn't work. Then we tried baby food in the jar, and that didn't work either. Meanwhile, all my vitals improved. My A1C went from 10.7 to 7.4, my creatine level improved as well as my blood pressure; all of this occurred in just a couple of months. I stopped taking all medications, and God did that. Every measurement, when they took my blood work at the VA hospital, showed improvement. Now how do you explain that? I never slept a full night. God would get me up. My mouth would be so dry, and my throat would close up, and while I was up, He said, *"Go and write I have something else to tell you about Forced to Focus."* That was every single day and night. That was the process I went through. I didn't get physically tired although it took a toll on me. I didn't have a high energy level some days, and sometimes, I felt like doing more things than others. So that I didn't think about time and my condition, God kept me doing things; and that hasn't changed.

At first, I was told I would have 30 radiation treatments, but by the third opinion, I needed 33 radiation treatments. I'm like *three more. Why do I need three more*? Everything that they told me would happen actually happened, but nothing happened right away, so I was like, oh, *I got this,* until things started happening. I asked what I should expect, and I was told my face would get dark and it would be 5-6 weeks before I would get my taste back. My last radiation treatment was on September 17, 2021, and I wanted to eat the next day. No food worked, so the Lord told me to try the broth. My 3-4 meals per day became chicken and beef broth. I would just put it in a bowl and warm it up because I still couldn't eat solid food. As I tackled that part of my journey, God said, I am continuously blessing you, but if I bless you now to be able to eat immediately, you will lose your focus, and I'm not done with you yet!

What are you missing? What is it that you don't have that you want? I tell Him that I just want more of Him. Everyday...

He wants me to know that it is Him, and He told me that He does not want me to be comfortable. There are things that I am praying for, and there cannot be any distraction between my prayers to Him and strength to wait on Him. He is a Deliverer!

I knew that God wanted me to endure this journey because He had given me the strength to do so. I experienced physical changes from the radiation, like the burning of my hair follicles and facial nerves. Today, as I write this, my face is hard and still tender to the touch. When I yawn, it hurts because I can't open my mouth, the pain comes and goes, and my hearing is still compromised. But my wife continues to encourage me, speaking words of life and healing. With each physical challenge my thoughts remained the same, *I know I have to pray now.* God can't release me because He is not finished with me yet, so I've come to accept that.

Chapter Three

Our Forever Walk – A wife's perspective

It was in August of 1970 that Ron and I met. He was a Junior Executive at Blue Cross and Blue Shield of Michigan in Downtown Detroit, and I worked at a small chic Boutique on Monroe Street in Downtown Detroit. One wonderful day, I saw my future walking down the street, and I thought he was the cutest man I had ever seen before in my young life. I was a seventeen-year-old high school senior, and I was fascinated by his strong, masculine build and looks. I thought to myself, *I'm going to get him*, and that was that. Well, not many days from the initial look and thought, I approached him and asked if he wanted my phone number—he said NO! That's when the challenge began, and the fight for his attention and love started.

Well after the 'No,' I began to pursue him like a bill collector, and he didn't have a safe place to put his feelings for me. After all, he was the only black junior executive that had my attention, and I was the only young hazel-eyed girl that he had met at the time. Fast-forward, after a four-day company trip to Chicago, he found himself missing me, and came back to Detroit to claim me as his wife. Now, that's a brief synopsis of our beginning.

Let me tell you about my husband. He adds to his employment credit, Director, Blue Cross/Blue Shield of Michigan, past President & CEO of The Detroit Urban League, Retired Police Commissioner, and Wayne County Chaplain. He became a Pastor of the Rose of Sharon Church of God in Christ and an Administrative Assistant to our late Bishop, John H. Sheard. In addition, we have two children and eight grandchildren, one son-in-law and one daughter-in-love. We have experienced a great deal of pleasure, disappointment, and challenges in our years of holy matrimony/marriage. However, I am a Bishop and First Lady's daughter, and I knew that our story would be different from most because I didn't marry a 'church man,' I sought a guy that liked to dance, finger pop, and drink wine—and I was indeed excited when he came into my life.

To be clear, I loved to party, drink wine and club. I was mad and very disappointed in my destiny. I knew without a doubt that my life as I once knew it was going to change and that I would certainly lose my battle with enjoying a life of partying with my husband!

Well Reader, please know that God has a great sense of humor, and that man didn't stay around long, only twelve of the 50 years we've been married. When Ron received that call from God Himself, my life turned upside down and topsy-turvy, and on May 9, 1983, our lives would never be the same. No more drinking, clubbing, dancing, lying, hanging out at our friends' homes, going to the movies, etc.; I'm sure you get the picture! God was getting us ready for our destiny. A future of praying, sacrifice, counseling, rebuilding married couples' lives, helping mentor teenage girls and boys, generating funds for scholarships to deserving college-aged young men and women, and providing food for the hungry and shelter for the homeless. Yes, God had a plan for us, and we were willing to obey His command.

Well, after many pastoral trials and tribulations, we were sailing right along, finding peace when we could and certainly weren't looking for drama; we had experienced enough of that during our early years of marriage and pastoral ministry. So, when the attack came, it was extremely subtle and unexpected—a lump on the side of my husband's face, right beside his ear. I was not extremely concerned about it because there was no pain, and he seemed not to be worried. But, after a few weeks, that passive attitude became one of concern after he went to the dentist and was advised that it wasn't a dental issue but internal in nature. I didn't show my fear or concern to my husband, but I was concerned about the lump and wanted it to disappear. So, he made the appointment with the Veterans Administration Hospital, and after careful examination, they determined it was a tumor. They told us that it wasn't a "big deal" because they felt that it was a benign tumor. They said they would remove it in a couple of weeks and that would be that…Well, you know that isn't the end of the story.

After a four-hour surgery and me preparing to take my husband home (the vows say for better or for worse), I was excited that once again, the storm that was prepared for us had indeed passed over, and we would again, just go home and it would be business as usual. We would go to the church and thank God for getting us through the surgery and continue with the ministry that God had placed us over. The four-hour surgery produced a malignant stage 3 cancerous tumor that was approximately 3 inches in diameter, and it was certainly the most repugnant looking thing I had ever seen.

Gone was the excitement of my birthday celebration—the flowers, romantic dinner, and beautiful car ride; not to mention, the masculine build, mustache, facial hair, and strong jawbone structure. IT WAS WAR AND PRAYER TIME. I immediately called the Cancer Treatment Center in Illinois for a second opinion, and after a four-day stay, they concurred with the diagnosis that the tumor was indeed in its 3rd stage and that the dreaded RADIATION would be needed to get rid of the cancer. SO, MY PRAYER JOURNEY BEGINS! For the next few months, I went into battle and locked my head and conversation around the fact that Ron had to live and not die to declare the works of the Lord, and I only spoke positive things in his presence: and kept negative people and situations away from him and his healing. Proverbs clearly states that, "The tongue has the power of life and death, and those who love it will eat its fruit." So, I began to consult God and made it my business to eat light and pray heavily.

Every day, I went to treatment with my husband and waited while they placed the device on his body. I watched his weight decrease, and the doctors and nurses looked in astonishment when he didn't give in to the radiation and the terrible damage it normally causes. We experienced God in His Glory. After his 33rd treatment, they rang the bell, indicating the cancer was eradicated, and he had beat the challenge that was placed before us. They gave the treatment the glory; we gave the Glory to God. For it was Him that maintained Ron's peace while losing forty pounds. It was God that gave my husband the blessed assurance that He would deliver him out of the fiery furnace without being burned or smelling like smoke. Well, I can testify that God did what He assured my dear husband that He would do. The treatment only assured us that God was in control, and that while we went in the fiery furnace, God brought us out. After many days of me watching God do His work on my dearly beloved soul mate, I am convinced that God called us, and that

He will allow the Saints to be placed in a situation that requires you to focus on Him and Him alone—when man can't help you, God will. Amen?

Chapter Four

The Mask

The Treatment Process

Let's recap the "Journey so far"

- I noticed the lump in April 2021–
- Diagnosed as a Warthin Tumor and had it surgically removed in May 2021.
- Received the Pathologist Report of Stage 3 cancer in June 2021.
- Obtained a 2nd opinion in July 2021 – (Stage 3 Cancer – 30 radiation treatment recommended, later changed to 33).
- Prepared for radiation treatment in July 2021.
- Started treatments – August 3, 2021.

Now, allow me to share the process with you. In the consultation with the oncology team, I was informed that I would have 33 radiation treatments Monday thru Friday, until completion. I was prepared for the treatment by the creation of a face, shoulder-chest mask that would keep me immobilized while taking the treatment. I had "no clue" what that would entail, however; I would soon find out. The mask was the "new technology" for radiation treatment that would fit over my face, shoulders, and upper part of my chest. The mask would be bolted to the rotating table much like the one when cat scans and MRIs are required. My feet would be bound by an elastic band so that I would be perfectly still during the treatment. The mask fit so tight that my eyes and mouth were shut, and I was told that if I was in any distress, "just raise your hands" and the Oncology radiation technician would respond – (of course I had to preach that: *Just Raise your hands*).

I was scheduled for the treatment at 9:45 am Monday-Friday. It was during my first treatment, bound without movement, bound without the ability to open my mouth or eyes –bound by almost the impossibility to even swallow that I had to call on the name of the Lord and He was there. He spoke to me in the spirit, "*Forced to Focus*". I had no choice. I real ized that I couldn't make it without Him. Each day, I prayed before each treatment, during each treatment and I thanked Him profusely after each treatment. Linda and I had a "routine" we followed. She was with me every day, every step of the way, every consultation with the staff and every treatment. She did not miss one of the 33 treatments. Her support was unmeasurable.

The daily routine was to get dressed, go to the VA., greet the Covid 19 screeners with a smile and words of encouragement, arrive early – (before 9:45 AM) be ready, without hesitation take the treatment. Linda was the only one who came daily – the other patients mostly came alone. Each day I became stronger spiritually because I was "*Forced to Focus*" on Him.

Let me share with you – no matter what you're going through, I promise you that if you put your trust and faith in him, He will see you through.

As the process continued, my taste for food began to disappear. The radiation, while "burning away" the malignant cancer, also temporarily "destroyed" my ability to taste and digest solid food. I ate my last solid food around the middle of August during our 50th wedding anniversary. From then on, it was a liquid diet only. Of course, I began to lose weight. I started the preliminary exam at 190 lbs. from there – 184, 180, 175, 170, all the way to 165 by the time we completed the 33rd treatment. The weight loss continued for another 30 days.

The staff and nurse were so concerned, and compassionate. The nurse stated that many become so weakened by the weight loss that wheelchairs are required for them. Well, I can tell you that God granted me strength. I never wavered, never stumbled, and never showed any signs that I could not withstand the effects of the radiation. *To God Be the Glory*, not me, it was all Him. In following the liquid diet, I tried Glycerna, protein supplements, Jello, frozen fruit popsicles, baby food (yes baby food) all to no avail. My daily intake was less than 500 calories daily. Compared to the American Medical Association nutritional guidelines, 2000 calories daily for men and 2500 daily for women, but God was able to sustain my body on less than 500 calories daily. The process continued without interruptions, and I continued the treatments; only 15 left, only 10 left – until the last week, 5, 4, 3, 2, 1. Hallelujah thanks and praises to God; this stage of the process was finally over. Allow me to pause for a moment to tell you the favor God gave me with the staff. They showed me great respect, concern, compassion, and comfort. From time to time, they would even ask "what did I preach" as it pertained to the treatments.

On Friday, September 17th – at approximately 10:00 am the oncology staff rung the bell symbolizing that I successfully completed my course. The implication was that I was cancer free. Of course, I was grateful and thankful; however, I had His blessed assurance that I would be *healed, delivered, and set free* from all the cancer in my body. To Him be all the Glory, Honor and Praise. I told the Medical Team both in the Cancer Center of America in Illinois and the team at the VA. I have confidence in medical science and abiding Faith in God. Finally, as this phase of the process ended, the Lord gave me the strength to officiate at the wedding celebration of our oldest granddaughter a hot and beautiful day. As I stood there in my white robe, I was still "*Forced to Focus*" needing Him to get me through the day and He did. Once again: To God Be the Glory.

Chapter Five

Blessed During the Journey

The Lord gave a word of encouragement for me to share with the world. He said, "Count your blessings, not your disappointments." That of course was very profound as we, the people of God, tend to allow the enemy to infiltrate our "spiritual space" and distract us from all the blessings that God has bestowed on us and simply concentrate on our trials, tribulations, disappointments, and dark days. Well, it was during the process discussed in Chapter 4 that He once again reminded me to count my blessings not my disappointments. He forced me to focus on how blessed I was in spite of the cancer. Here's what He spoke into my spirit: *"My servant, know that I've not allowed the cancer to spread – There has been no manifestation of the cancer in your mouth. (As the oncologist checked weekly for evidence of radiation burn or sores) There has been no sore throat from the radiation – I have blessed your body to survive-prosper through 500 calories daily. You have survived on a liquid diet and not solid food.* He gave me the scripture to support this, Matthew 4:4 "It is written, man shall not live by bread alone, but by every word that proceedeth out of the mouth of God."

He continued, *"You have not taken any pain medication over the last 15 radiation treatments. Your A1C was lowered from 10:7 to 7:4 in the last 30 plus days. And if that's not enough, I blessed you with those who called you with words of encouragement and anointed prayers. Some have even blessed you financially. They have traveled 200 miles to visit and fellowship. And just as I blessed the children of Israel in the wilderness with manna from heaven; (Exodus 16:1-36, and Numbers 11:1-9) I fed you a liquid diet including V8 juices, chicken, and beef broth and "Pot licker" – from collard and mustard greens. You are blessed and the best is yet to come."* This reminder from the Lord was so necessary because I needed to feel His presence. It didn't mean that I had lost faith, it simply meant that

I was "going through." The manifestation of the cancer is and was real but so was and is God's promises. He promised that He would heal my body. I know that He is able to perform that which He will. In addition, He has given me the strength to keep standing. I don't look sick, I don't feel sick, I don't act sick, because I'm not sick. All the praise, honor, glory, and reverence are His. And if all of the above is not enough, I'm so very grateful and thankful that He chose me for this journey. I'm glad He trusts me enough to know that I have not and will not stop praising, worshipping, and glorifying Him in the midst of this cancer journey.

I'm becoming closer to Him. I know Him better and more personally. I now can better understand the old gospel hymn, "You'll understand it better, by and by." So be encouraged, be strong, stay focused on our Lord and Savior Jesus Christ, who is the Author and Finisher of our faith. Stay focused on the only one that can deliver us from all of our trials and tribulations. Remember this, Psalm 34:19 says, "Many are the afflictions of the righteous: But the Lord delivereth him out of them all"— and in song, we have His blessed assurance. We place all our hopes on God and His word. That's why I am Blessed in the midst of this cancer journey."

Chapter Six

It Ain't Over

When I completed the treatments; I was ready to somewhat resume eating solid food, returning to a few of my routine activities, maybe even to some extent, "business as usual," of which I would routinely preach against. Those thoughts were soon driven away as the Lord spoke to me, "It ain't over, I have further need of you to remain focused; and yet again, I was "*Forced to Focus*". He reminded me that this cancer journey was all to His glory and the least I could do for all of His benefits toward me. (Psalm 116:12) It's what I'm "rendering," and my show of gratitude.

You see, there are some powerful prayer requests I have before Him. There are some "strongholds" that must be destroyed and in order for that to happen, the Lord must be able to speak to me with clarity. He must have my undivided attention. He also said, *"For what you're asking and seeking you must continue to fast and pray—no solid food.* (Matthew 17:21), "Howbeit this kind goeth not out but by prayer and fasting" And I heard His words loud and clear just as I was thinking about smothered pork chops, rice, mushroom gravy, greens, yams, ribs, potato salad, black eyed peas, corn bread, a corned beef sandwich with chips, etc., not to mention peach cobbler. Again, He reminded me that man couldn't live by bread alone. (Matthew 4:4)

He needed me to remain focused on Him and not solid food. He was sustaining me just enough to fulfill His purpose. This was yet another "lesson" for me to learn. I continued the liquid diet and kept my focus on the important aspects of this cancer journey. To His glory and to my desire for victory and the destruction of strongholds, that the Rose of Sharon members were experiencing, as well as my extended family, I was "*Forced to focus*". We need to understand as I now do, that if we are serious of becoming more like Christ; if we are serious about being used by Him; if we are serious about becoming and realizing victory in this confused, angry divided world, we must from time to time hide ourselves away in quiet, solitude so that we can hear from Him. We, likewise, must deny the flesh because worldly pursuits can and will become a distraction, as we seek the Lord's direction.

It ain't over simply means Satan continues to seek whom he may devour, (Peter 5:8) "Be sober, be vigilant because your adversary the devil, as the roaring lion, walketh about, seeking whom he may devour"; therefore, you have to be sober minded and alert in order for us to be watchful and clear in our thinking. Praying, and fasting is a necessity for all BELIEVERS.

Another 'nugget' that I teach and wish to share with you is this:

There are three times when we are most vulnerable from the enemies' attacks.

1.) When we have prayed for such a long time, it seems as though heaven has closed its ears and doesn't hear us.
2.) When we get tired of praying and give up, just before we receive our deliverance, we act too soon just or too late.

3.) Right after we have been blessed, our prayer (s) answered, we are rejoicing and happy and we "Let our spiritual guard down." We stop praying and fasting for the moment and then comes the "sucker punch" and an attack comes from out of nowhere.

I'm sure you've experienced one if not all of these situations. The way to avoid them is to recognize that you must stay focused. Luke 18:1 says, "stay alert, prayerful and pray without ceasing." I Thessalonians 5:17 says, "Always pray and not to faint." Likewise, Matthew 26:41 says, "Watch and pray." So, It ain't over, but He's blessed me to be better prepared as this cancer journey continues. You see, the enemy has come to me saying, "You'll never eat solid food again; the cancer is not gone, it will return soon." Since I know the "Devil is a liar." (John 8:44 AMP Version) I stand on the One who is the Truth – (St. John 8:31-32), I am victorious-in Him, I'm so glad that the Lord is yet leading me and placing me in situations where I am "*Forced to Focus*".

Chapter Seven

I'm Still Standing

As I have maneuvered thus far through this cancer journey, it has been made absolutely and abundantly clear that all I've been through, I'm still standing. What the Lord is doing and by faith what I believe He's going to do is overwhelming. I'm still standing in spite of going through 33 radiation treatments. I'm still standing after functioning on a liquid diet of less than 500 calories daily. I'm still standing having lost approximately 40 lbs. (Haven't been this weight, 150 lbs. since 1965). I'm still standing because my assignment is not over, and my work is not done.

I'm still standing all to His glory. I'm still standing because I was "*Forced to Focus*" on Him and Him alone. I'm still standing because God wants to use me as an example for others to see that He is yet in control.

He is sending a message, the message to all believers to return and non-believers alike to accept Him. He has reminded us that we can't fix the problems of this world until and unless we heed the Word found in II Chronicles 7:14, "If my people, which are called by my name shall humble themselves and pray, and seek my face, and turn from their wicked ways; then will I hear from Heaven and will forgive their sin and will heal their land." He is making it clear that if we trust in the Lord and lean not unto our own understanding. In all thy ways acknowledge Him and He will direct thy path, that the problems of this world will be fixed. I'm still standing because He's directing my path.

God has a powerful "track record."

- Look what He did for Job. (Job: 42) Job lost everything, and battled terribly in his body, yet he stood in faith, and saw the salvation of the Lord. God gave him double all that he lost.
- Look what He did for David (Psalms 142) David cried unto the Lord and He answered.

- Look what He did for Esther (Esther 1) He made her a queen and used her to save many.
- Look what He did for Paul (Acts 9:1-19) He changed Paul's entire life. He turned a murderer into a Saint, and Paul wrote the majority of the New Testament.
- Look what He did for the three Hebrew Boys (Daniel 3:1-30) He kept them from being burned alive. In fact, they didn't even smell like smoke.

And then there's Jesus! And just think about what Jesus did for us, Hallelujah! There are so many more examples.

So now remember what He's done for you. Aren't you still standing? I'm still standing because of His strength, His power, His kindness, His mercy, His love, His favor, His healing virtue, and His will. The Lord found that He could trust me and that I'll praise Him no matter what!! So, lift up your hands, all of you that have your own personal testimony of how you're *still standing*. And those who have been knocked down by the weight of life's struggles, please be encouraged and believe in God. Get up, by faith! Rise and take your bed and walk. I'm still standing; We're still standing and for those that've been knocked down, we're praying that you will stand again.

Chapter Eight

Trust God

The Lord says in Psalm 32:8 "I will instruct (teach) Thee in the way which Thou shalt go: I will guide Thee with mine eye." This is a companion scripture to Proverbs 3:5-6 – "Trust in the Lord with all thine heart, lean not to thy own understanding. In all thy ways acknowledge Him and He shall direct thy path. By now, many of you know that I have been chosen by God to trust Him as never before. I was placed in a position that I had to lean on Him, depend on Him and obey His word.

God had a plan for me; Jeremiah 29:11 – "For I know the thoughts that I think toward you saith the Lord, thoughts of peace, and not of evil, to give you an expected end. Then shall you call upon me, and ye shall go and pray unto me, and I will hearken unto you." What a comfort it is to know that with God there are no "coincidences or accidents." God is a God of purpose, and destiny. He allowed Stage 3 cancer to infiltrate my body and disallowed it as He heals my body. I trusted Him to do so. I knew that He could; I believed that He would.

I'm bringing you this message to encourage you as you go through your own journey and life challenges, to absolutely trust God. Lean on Him, depend on Him and reach out to Him in Prayer. I'm convinced, as I meditate on His word day and night, that I'm on a special assignment all to His Glory and to strengthen my relationship with Him.

I would implore you to consider that perhaps our Lord and Savior Jesus Christ has a need for you. Take another look at your situation and instead of worry, anxiety, doubt, anger, fear, trust in the Lord with all thine heart and lean not to your own understanding. Believe that He is able to take you through your personal journey.

What has been your experience? Didn't He do it before? Didn't He hear you the last time? Don't you have testimony of past deliverances and second chances? Isaiah 53:1 says, "Who hath believed our report? And whom is the arm of the Lord revealed." So, this is not rhetorical; "Whose report do you believe?" I believe the report of the Lord. He is a healer, deliverer, and a very present help in times of trouble. I was sent to bring you this message of hope. This message is to give you strength and to invite you to return unto Him, the Author and Finisher of our faith. This message is to comfort you and to make some sense out of the demonic influences and craziness that exists everywhere. This message is to let you know that God is yet in control. This message is to let you know that because He is in control, victory is yours for the asking!

I've shared with you that medical science has confirmed that Stage 3 cancer will be eradicated with 33 radiation treatments and "probably" won't return (a reasonable prognosis), but yet, Whose report do I believe? I believe in the Lord who is able to completely heal my body. I don't ask how or when; I just believe that He will! It's our faith that pleases Him. What are you believing God for?

Now let's take a moment to remember.

- Do you remember Hezekiah's testimony when he was told that he was going to die? Hezekiah prayed tearfully to God and God said," I have heard your prayer and have seen your tears; I will heal you." (Read 1 Kings 20) 15 years were added to his life.
- Do you remember Abraham and Sarah's testimony? How long they waited for the promise of God that they would become parents when she was 90 years old, and Abraham would be the Father at 100. Medical science would say that's impossible but "Whose report will you believe?" (Genesis 21:1-7)
- Do you remember the testimony of the woman who suffered 12 long years with a health challenge that the Doctor's couldn't heal? But the Bible says at Mark 5:27, "She heard about Jesus," and you know the rest.

Now, I have my own testimonies of how I remember God's report that I was going to be healed.

- First, Medical Science said, "It was caught in time." God said to me: Go tell medical science that you have a problem. They didn't know it, I did.

- Second, Medical Science said after the cat scan the cancer didn't spread. God said, "I stopped it – as a down payment on your healing."
- Third, Medical science said it's a rare form of cancer that can be treated. God said "I kept it simple just to get your attention all for my purpose and glory. It could have been so much worse. I even put it in a good location to be treated." Whose report will you believe, I believe the report of the Lord. I'm a chosen vessel blessed to carry out God's purpose.
- Fourth, Medical Science has prescribed organic, medication and a wholesome diet. God said to take a daily dose of prayer, supplemented by a steady diet of His word. If I don't see immediate results, "double up." Whose report will you believe? I believe the report of the Lord; trust Him and watch Him work.

"Comforting words in times like these"

Psalms 9:9-10 states, "The Lord also will be a refuge for the oppressed, a refuge in times of trouble. 10.) And those that know thy name will put their trust in thee." Psalm 46:1 says, "God is our refuge and strength, a very present help in trouble."

What a world, "A ball of confusion" as sung by the Motown recording group—The Temptations. So much going on that is out of our control; undrinkable, lead poisoned water in too many of our communities with long term health problems. Drainage systems that can't han-dle the rainstorms, backing up and causing major dam-age and destruction to homes and personal items. It seems as though the Municipal government we depend upon either can't or won't fix the problem. Injustices continue without regard for the sanctity of life and any compassion for humanity. Drugs that were once considered criminal and destructive are now acceptable as revenue driving the economy across the nation. Our elected officials who are supposed to represent us far too often, have their own agenda. Billions spent on space exploration, but what does that matter in communities that have unclean water, unsafe living conditions, far reaching health issues and poor housing and all sorts of violence in their/our communities. There are over 200 Christian denominations in the US and 45,000 all over the world. Some 380,000 churches in the US—not including Synagogues and Mosques and we still hate each other.

Now, add to all of the above our daily struggles, trials, hard times, sleepless nights, and stressful days.

Consider the everyday challenge of trying "to make ends meet." Trying to simply create a useful life with some sense of peace. It can become an overwhelming task. We want to quit and are ready to give up. We become stressed and depressed. Some even take or want to take their own lives and nothing seems to work so life becomes meaningless and so on. However, I am commanded by the Lord to invite you to read the Word for today; believe it, stand on it, live by it, and put your faith and hope in Him. God is our refuge, "A safe place" and strength. (Psalm 46:1) Are you a witness that He is your strength, and a very present help in times of trouble? We used to say, "He's an on-time God! Yes, He is," and the text goes on to say, do not fear no matter what.

No matter how dark it looks, bad it gets, hopeless it seems, and depressed we feel: God got our back and there's more.

Psalm 9:9-10 Reassures us that the Lord is also a refuge for the oppressed (abused by those who exercise control over us) And in times of trouble, how comforting it is to know that they who know His name will trust Him. (Proverbs 3:5-6) Trust God and Him alone for He has not forsaken them that seek Him. Remember that last time we needed Him, didn't he come through for us? Yes, He did. Not only does He know, but He also cares.

For further comfort–

Psalm 23 – "The Lord is my shepherd; I shall not want - He makes me to lie down in green pastures. He leadeth me beside the still waters He restoreth my soul. He leadeth me in the paths of righteousness for his name's sake. Yea, though I walk through the valley of the shadow of death I will fear no evil for thou art with me Thy rod and thy staff they comfort me. Thou preparest a table before me in the presence of my enemies: thou anointest my head with oil, my cup runneth over. Surely goodness and mercy shall follow me all the days of my life: and I will dwell in the House of the Lord forever." Ain't that comfort in times like this?" Trust God and pray.

Food for Thought

Exodus 15:22-6 – "So Moses brought Israel from the Red Sea and they went out into the wilderness of Shur; and they went three days in the wilderness, and found no water, 23.) And when they came to Marah, they and they went three days in the wilderness, and found no water, 23.) And when they came to Marah, they could not drink of the waters of Marah for they were bitter therefore the name of it was called Mara 24.) And the people murmured against Moses saying, "what shall we drink." 25.) And he cried unto the Lord: and the Lord shewed him a tree, which when he had cast into the waters, the waters were made sweet: There he made for them a statue and an ordinance and there He proved to them and said, "If thou wilt diligently hearken to the voice of the Lord thy God, and wilt do that which is right in His sight, and wilt give ear to his commandments and keep all His statutes, I will put none of these diseases upon thee which I have brought upon the Egyptians, For I am the Lord that healeth thee."

God's promise comes with strings attached
It's a small price to pay

This message is intended to encourage you, to lift you up and get you to remember how He got you through your most recent crisis. He especially wants you to remember your last blessing or the last time you were delivered from a bad situation; A dark moment, if you will. We must continue to remember. The enemy doesn't want us to focus on how awesome God is—but rather focus on the negative. Do you remember the last time, the most recent time you were delivered, healed, and set free? On the other hand, do you remember when you thought, finally everything was *"going your way."* Or you could *"see the light of day."* Have you ever said, *"I'm making the ends meet, and now I can get some peace." Or, "Finally, I've overcome that dark situation."* Then comes another attack.

Do you remember how helpless and hopeless you felt? Do you remember what you said and most importantly how it affected your relationship with the Lord? Did your faith waiver? Did you ask Him, "How long must I suffer? What did I do wrong? Why have you abandoned me?" Did you call God into question?

Here are some examples of God moving in the lives of His people:

- God has delivered the children of Israel from the bondage of Pharoah
- Pharoah and his entire army are all dead
- The people are rejoicing, singing declaring how great was their victory

Miriam, the Prophetess, the sister of Aaron, took a timbrell in her hand and all the women went out after her with timbrels and with dancers.

Now it gets interesting….

- Moses took the people into the wilderness of Shur – they found no water (3 days)
- And when they found water, it was bitter (contamination – not fit to drink)
- And the people start to complain to Moses saying: "What shall we drink?"
- Moses cried out unto the Lord –
- A tree in the water-made it sweet.

Now comes the really good part that serves as the foundation for this lesson/message….

- Strings attached – one or more conditions, restrictions, obligations, or arrangements that must be met for one to attain something they desire. Help me to say "strings attached" what were these "strings" – His voice speaks!!
    - Do right in the sight of God
    - Give ear to His commandments
    - Keep his statues

That's it – and if you do these things, I promise I will put none of these diseases upon thee, which I have brought upon the Egyptians for I am the Lord that healeth thee.

What a small price to pay....

- Do right in His sight
- Just hear, pay attention to what He has to say
- Keep His statues

Allow me to simplify – Read, study, and obey the Word of God

II Chronicles 7:14 – "Some strings attached" If my people - which are called by my name – shall humble, themselves, and pray and seek my face, and turn from their wicked ways. Then will I hear from Heaven and will forgive their sin and will heal the Lord. It's a small price to pay, trust God and Pray.

Chapter Nine

A Spiritual Taste test

Psalm 34:8 - *"O' taste and see that the Lord is good; blessed is the man that trusted in Him."*

About the time I had radiation treatment number 15, I experienced a complete loss of taste, with no desire to eat solid food. While my focus was on satisfying "the flesh," I knew that, in reality, it was "spiritual food that I would need in order to get through the cancer journey." In the midst of my ordeal, the Lord spoke to me in the Spirit leading me to the text at Psalm 34: 8. I had repeated it many times in my nearly 30 years of pastoring, but now it had a more profound impact on my life. There is a saying; "You can't get there until you get there." It took this "test" to get me there. The text wants us to literally taste, sample and try Him. In essence, give God a chance. We've tried to reason, analyze, and figure it out using the world's methods to no avail. So, let's try Him.

Don't simply take my word for it. Try Him for yourself. Get up close and personal. Stop trying to figure it out and fix it on your own. Trust him and watch him work. To see implies that you have come into the knowledge and understanding that when you turn it over to Jesus, He'll make everything alright. You've watched Him work, and you can see clearly now. You were looking at your situation like trying to look into shallow water that was dark and murky. Now, the mud and debris settled to the bottom thus restoring its clarity. You can now see what others cannot because you're now looking through spiritual eyes and not carnal.

I Peter 2:2-3 says, "As Newborn babes, desire the sincere milk of the word that ye may grow thereby: If so be ye have tasted that the Lord is gracious." Psalm 145:8 says, "The Lord is gracious and merciful: slow to anger and great in loving kindness."

Now take a look at how this scripture ends, *Blessed is the man that trusteth in Him. I am a witness when you taste and see, you'll find your faith will grow your confidence in Him and will cause you to get closer to Him. Your foundation will become stronger, you will become unmovable and unshakable in your commitment. And you'll understand it better "by and by."* Ain't nobody like Jesus!!

Triumph over Trauma

There are times when we experience trauma, and face a crisis, that the only one that we can go to is the Lord. I believe that God allows some circumstances to overtake us so we can come to Him and Him alone. And by doing so, we realize just how great God is. "*Forced to Focus*" parallel's Paul's dilemma and testimony. "A thorn in the Flesh," kept Him humble and moved on Him to see God. David was moved to bless the Lord at all times and to acknowledge that his praise will continually be in his mouth. So, then we must focus on God and not ourselves. Focusing on Him helps to put everything in perspective.

Focusing on Him with our minds, body, and soul we limit and eliminate self-pity and doubt. We come to realize that His grace is sufficient. When we focus on Him and spend time with Him in prayer, quiet meditation, fasting and studying His word, we become fully aware of just how great He is. So, then as we go through our daily trials and tribulation, our darkest period in our lives, and other traumatic experiences – we stop for a moment to reflect on "counting our blessings and not our disappointments."

Taking this a step further, it's no wonder I will bless the Lord at all times and pray that you who are reading will do the same. Bless the Lord at all times and then be found praising the Lord continually. Praise in our mouth meaning we are ready to praise Him right now! We confuse the enemy when we praise God. The enemy's job is to kill, steal and destroy but yet we are still blessing and praising the Lord.

I continue to trust God because I've researched His past and the powerful work He's done.

He parted the red sea,

He brought down the Jericho wall,

He protected and delivered the Hebrew Boys in the furnace,

He fed the multitude with 2 fish, and 5 loaves of bread,

He protected Daniel in the Lion's Den,

He died and rose on the 3rd day and returned to His father.

But most important of all, He saved, sanctified, and filled me with the Baptism of His Holy Spirit and now as I go through my cancer journey, I've come to know that I must bless Him at all times and praise Him continually. Since He did all that and more, He can do it for me. Won't you join me with a moment of praise no matter what we're going through. It's a blessing when we are "*Forced to Focus.*" This is my way of knowing that God has His "eyes" on me; it's personal. It means He loves me. Knowing in advance what I'm going to experience, means that as I focus on Him and count my blessings, it's important that I give Him all the glory, honor, praise, and reverence – all the time.

Chapter Ten

The Battle is the Lord's

II Chronicles 20:1-30 *"You don't have to wait until the battle is over; you can shout now."*

My process of studying and preparing my message for church was interrupted by a call from Sis. Meaghan Madison, our choir director and praise team leader. During the conversation, she asked was I going to have a special service celebrating and praising God for my healing of cancer, after the last of 33 radiation treatments? As I thought about that, the Holy Ghost spoke to me and said, "You don't have to wait until the battle is over, you can shout now."

Here are some bullet points from the story in II Chronicles:

- The enemies-MOAB and Ammon and the inhabitants of MT. Seir.
- To: King Jehoshaphat – "You are surrounded by your enemies."
    - Jehoshaphat was frightened and prayed to the Lord for guidance
    - Time to fast
    - He prayed with a purpose!!
    - God sent Jahaziel – (son of Zechariah) to King Jehoshaphat". Don't be discouraged or afraid to face the enemy. The battle is God's – not yours.
    - Just get into position-right place, right time, right attitude
    - King Jehoshaphat in verse 20 – "Put your trust in the Lord your God and stand firm.
    - The King ordered some of the musicians to put on the robes (sacred) and march ahead of the army-singing. "Praise the Lord!! His love is eternal.
    - When they began to sing – The Lord threw the invading armies into a panic, and they began to attack each other.

Sometimes God will fight the actual battle through us, and at other times, He will simply tell us to hold our positions, stand still and do nothing except to pray and trust Him. Watch Him intervene and demonstrate His awesome power when He decides to defeat the enemy personally Protecting us as only, He can. At any rate, "we don't have to wait until the battle is over, we can shout now!" And "shout" is what I did. I danced until I could barely breathe and stand upright. I couldn't wait any longer to show my faith and trust in Him.

"It's the least I can do"

One of my favorite scriptures is Psalms 116:12, "What shall I render unto the Lord for all His benefits towards me?" (How can I repay the Lord for all of His blessings). As I have shared with you in the past "We should count our blessings and not our disappointments." I began to focus my attention once again towards How blessed I am. I was moved to this spiritual place as we are in our room at The Cancer Treatment Center of America – in Zion, Illinois, about an hour north of Chicago. I thought about His blessings and benefits.

He has blessed me materially and spiritually with favor and rewarded my faith. He has shown me the magnificence of His mercy. I am the recipient of His redemption and reconciliation. I realize that medical science can treat and cure my cancer but only God can heal and deliver! He has brought me into the presence of medical experts in every phase of cancer. I know my Lord and Savior need to do nothing more than to "speak to it" and it's gone. All of my hope and faith are in Jesus, the Messiah, my Savior. I have some prayers before the Lord more important to me, than to be healed of cancer. And you, the members of the Rose, my family and for those who have reached out to me to "stand in the gap" on your behalf.

It's my prayer that...

- Those of you who have knowingly walked away from God-please return.
- Those who seek forgiveness-reach out to those whom you have harmed and ask in all humility and sincerity for their forgiveness.
- Those who have been harmed – forgive those who did it and perhaps have not acknowledged it.
- Families are reunited not just for a "reunion", but because of the great work that can be accomplished when we all work together in love and unity and to please Him.
- Those who have almost given up on life please rise up, by praying, fasting, and trusting Him again.

What Shall I Render? – I can praise Him no matter what. I can show my gratitude by serving Him and Him alone. I can open up my bowels of mercy to those He sends into my life. I can testify and witness of His awesome power. I can willingly obey, worship, and glorify His very name. I can stand ready to do whatever He desires for me to do. What shall I render unto the Lord for all of His benefits toward me; all of the above, all the days of my life? What will *you* render? Please give back to the Lord for all that He's done and will do for you. If nothing else, simply tell the Lord THANK YOU!

End Notes: Warthin Tumor

W**arthin tumor** is a benign tumor of the salivary gland. The first symptom is usually a painless, slow-growing bump in front of the ear, on the bottom of the mouth, or under the chin. Warthin tumors may increase in size over time, but few become cancerous. Though the cause is currently unknown, smoking is believed to increase the chance of developing Warthin tumor. Treatment may consist of surgery to remove the tumor or careful observation to watch for changes in the tumor over time.

Symptoms

Warthin tumor is a benign (noncancerous) tumor of the salivary glands. They most commonly arise in the parotid glands, the largest salivary glands which are located in each cheek above the jaw in front of the ears. Approximately 5-14% of cases are bilateral and 12-20% of affected people experience multicentric (more than one tumor which formed separately from one another) disease. The first symptom is usually a firm, painless bump. Without treatment, the swelling may gradually increase overtime which can cause facial nerve palsy (difficulty moving one side of the face).

Cause

The exact underlying cause of Warthin tumor is currently unknown. However, smoking is thought to increase the risk of developing the tumor. Some studies suggest that radiation exposure and autoimmune disorders may also be associated with Warthin tumor.

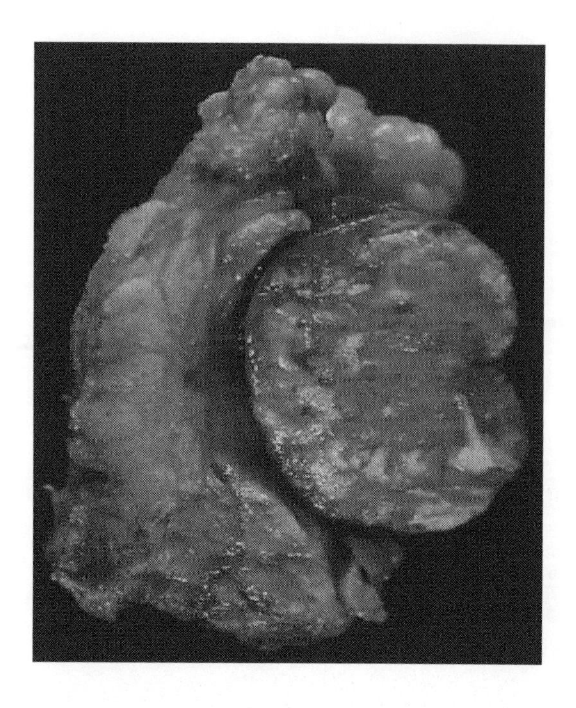

Parotid Gland

The **parotid gland** is a major salivary gland in many animals. In humans, the two parotid glands are present on either side of the mouth and in front of both ears. They are the largest of the salivary glands. Each parotid is wrapped around the mandibular ramus, and secretes serous saliva through the parotid duct into the mouth, to facilitate mastication and swallowing and to begin the digestion of starches. There are also two other types of salivary glands; they are submandibular and sublingual glands.[1] Sometimes **accessory parotid glands** are found close to the main parotid glands.

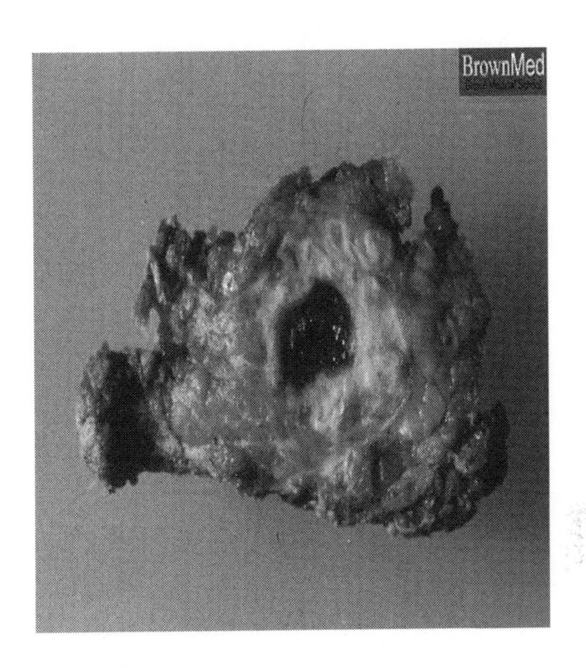

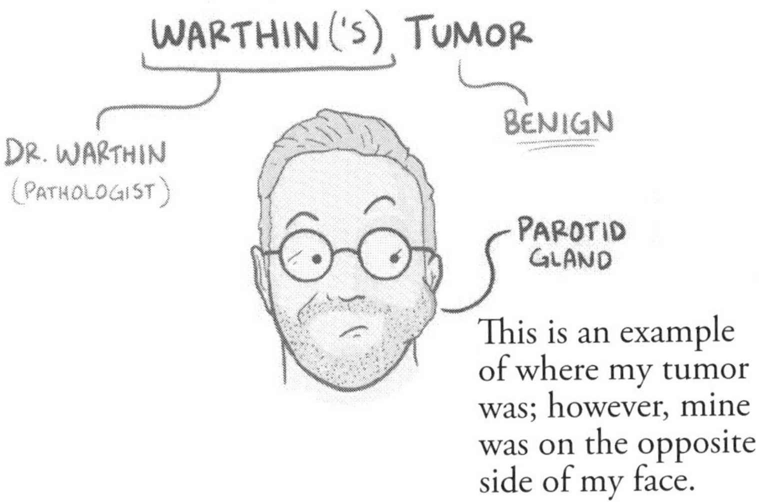

This is an example of where my tumor was; however, mine was on the opposite side of my face.

Reference:

Leviticus 18:5 - Commentary, explanation and study verse https://www.bibliaplus.org/en/leviticus/18/5

https://en.wikipedia.org/wiki/Parotid_gland

ACKNOWLEDGMENTS

I am so very thankful for the following persons who contributed to the completion of this project. They, through their understanding of how much "*Forced to Focus*," means to me, was the driving catalyst, ever encouraging me to keep on until the finish line was reached.

Not in order of importance – for all their efforts were necessary.

- Missy Charise Carter, Rose of Sharon Office Administrator – typed the entire manuscript at least three times.
- Regina Coleman, Kendra Ford and Zequetta Hall whose comments and insight were so valuable.

- The Coaching Team, Dr. Latonya Garth & Dr. Tara Tucker who really "took over" the project providing critical advice, council, and direction.
- My granddaughter, Hunter Simone Griffin, who was my "tech" advisor.
- The staff at the Cancer Treatment Center of America; located in Zion, Illinois.
- The John Dingell Jr. VA oncology team of Detroit.

The Launch Team: Elder Ronald H. Griffin, Lora Lewis, Regina Coleman, Dr's Garth and Tucker, Cliff Stovall who encouraged me daily. Now, last but impossible to be the least, Linda F. Griffin who not only inspired me continuously but actually was responsible for Chapter 3 of the book. It would be remiss of me if I did not acknowledge those who prayed for me during this journey both clergy and non-clergy alike. To mention them individually would lead me to forget anyone of them which I dare not do. I continue to feel the power of their prayers. What they did for me will never be forgotten.

About the Author

PASTOR RONALD L. GRIFFIN

On January 26, 1992, Pastor Ronald L. Griffin was installed as the second Pastor of the Rose of Sharon Church of God in Christ. His formative years were rooted in the loving discipline and spiritual guidance, he received from his parents, Vivian and Richard Clowney, and the Church of God in Christ

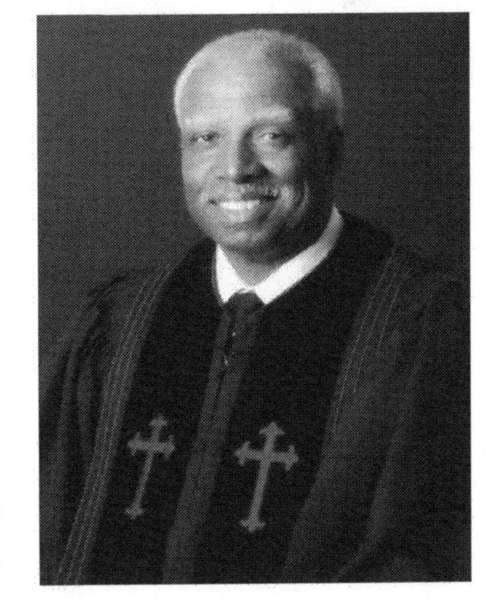

under the leadership of Bishops, Elders, and Mothers of the Church. Most significantly, in later years, his late father-in-law, Bishop Willie LeRoy Harris, and his late mother-in-law, Ima Harris, directed his theological formation and Christian thinking.

Pastor Griffin is a graduate of Southwestern High School and earned his Bachelor of General Studies degree with distinction from Wayne State University in 1980. The countless number of conferences, seminars, and workshops he attended further enhanced his leadership skills and training. For nearly 26 years, Pastor Griffin was employed at Blue Cross Blue Shield of Michigan in leadership/executive positions and was responsible for several key operations and hundreds of employees. Prior to devoting all of his time to his Pastoral Ministry, Pastor Griffin was President and Chief Executive Officer of the Detroit Urban League. In that capacity, he revitalized community programs and their relationship with other community organizations.

As added testimony to his leadership skills, his character, and his commitment to being God's servant, Pastor Griffin has received many commendations and has served on a number of community boards, some of which are:

- Past Vice Chair & Chair Detroit Board of Police Commissioner - 2008-2010
- Recipient of Certificate of Recognition from Chief of Police, Detroit Police Department in July 2002
- Recipient of Spirit of Detroit Award from Detroit City Council, July 2002
- Past Chairman of Public Relations and current member of the Executive Board, First Ecclesiastical Jurisdiction of Michigan Southwest
- Chairman of Superintendents, First Ecclesiastical Jurisdiction Michigan Southwest
- Member of the Care Corps - Wayne County Sheriff Chaplain
- Past member of the Business Education Alliance, an affiliate of the Detroit Chamber of Commerce
- Past member of the United Neighborhood Centers of America
- Past Board member, Historic Old Trinity Lutheran
- Lifetime member of NAACP
- Recipient of the Outstanding Young Man of America award in 1983
- Recipient of the YMCA Minority Achiever of the Year award in 1983

In July 1998, the late Bishop John H. Sheard, Jurisdictional Prelate, First Ecclesiastical, Michigan Southwest, appointed Pastor Griffin Superintendent. On August 28, 2011, at the 65th Annual Holy Convocation, Bishop John H. Sheard appointed Pastor Griffin as an Administrative-Assistant.

On a personal note, Pastor Griffin has been married 50 years to Linda F. Griffin. The Griffins have 2 Adult Children, 1 Daughter in Love and 1 Son in Love, 8 Grandchildren, 8 Godchildren and 6 God-Grandchildren.

Made in the USA
Monee, IL
27 March 2022